BOOK TITLE

HEALTHY ME:

The path to improved well-being

BY

Chilla Penzi

Introduction

You do not need to follow a diet of hunger! Healthy Me highlights the value of comprehending your metabolism and offers a nutritious strategy for losing weight. There are several approaches to raising your metabolism and well-being. Healthy Me demonstrates that improving one's level of energy and fitness is achievable. Rather than sacrificing your favorite meals, you should include more of them.

well, done. Healthy Me dispels myths about body fat and other weight-related concerns and provides information on the foods and activities that can help our bodies' recovery.

Chapter 1: Comprehending Body Fat

Chapter 2: Obesity's effects on health

Chapter 3: Maintaining a Sound Equilibrium

3.1: Consume a diet high in fruits, vegetables, and proteins and well-balanced.

3.2: Exercise for a minimum of 150 minutes per week.

3.3 Sleep for seven to nine hours per night.

Chapter 4: Mental well-being

4.1: Use self-massage, yoga, or meditation to unwind your body.

4.2: Make attainable objectives that you can strive for each day.

4.3: Engage in a joyful activity each day.

4.4: Acquire new knowledge.

4.5: Take care of your spiritual health.

Chapter 5: Balancing Work and Life

5.1: Create a budget for yourself.

5.2: Try to minimize the amount of work you accomplish at home.

5.3: Establish limits with your social groups, both at work and at home.

Chapter 1

Comprehending Body Fat

Fat is a necessary tissue in the body that performs several critical tasks, including operating as an organ in and of itself, storing energy for the body's key organs, and offering insulation and protection. Excess body fat can be present in even the thinnest individuals, according to research. Similar to how malignant tumors use blood vessels as a source of nutrition, this fat can expand and form blood vessels that supply it. the defensive mechanism known as "angiogenesis" in the body is in summary

You do not need to follow a diet of hunger! Healthy Me highlights the value of comprehending your metabolism and offers a nutritious strategy for losing weight. There are several approaches to raising your metabolism.

And well-being. Healthy Me demonstrates that improving one's level of energy and fitness is achievable.

Rather than sacrificing your favorite meals, you should include more of them.

 well, done. Healthy Me dispels myths about body fat and other

weight-related concerns and provides information on the foods and activities that can

our bodies' recovery.

urge to create and preserve blood vessels, and it is essential to overall health.

More than 70 illnesses, including cancer, can be caused by weakening angiogenesis.

Fortunately, the body's defenses against angiogenesis may be strengthened by over 100 nutrients, such as broccoli, ginseng, Turmeric, and soybeans. These diets prevent the formation of extraneous blood

These nutrients promote healthy circulation to aid in healing while preventing cancer cells from growing unwelcome blood vessels. This also applies to body fat's blood supply. The correct diet will stop the formation of extra blood vessels linked to the maintenance of fat.

Your body does not suffer from fat. Adipose stromal cells, or ASCs, and preadipocytes, two types of stem cells that are present in fat, are crucial for sustaining health.

Adipocytes are skilled in producing the fat cells that regulate metabolism, while ASCs are skilled in developing the blood vessels necessary for healthy fat tissue. When it comes to medical treatments like spinal cord regeneration, ASCs have demonstrated potential.

Trillions of bacteria, viruses, and fungi make up our body's microbiome, which affects wound healing, mental health, and general well-being. To improve your health and mental well-being. Think about other things besides fat if you want to be healthier. You need to support the growth of your microbiome as well, and you do this by not restricting the foods you eat. Along with other health advantages, a balanced and diversified microbiome that is fueled by plant-based diets and prebiotics helps to facilitate a more efficient metabolism.

Chapter 2

Obesity's effects on health

A complicated problem with several causes is obesity. It results from additional sugar; the body stores calories as fat. If you eat a lot of energy, especially in diets heavy in sugar and fat, and do not engage in physical exercise to expend all of the energy and much of the excess, the body will store energy as fat.

Obesity raises the risk of chronic inflammation and can have negative consequences for the immune system. The adipose tissue of obese individuals is home to a high concentration of immune cells known as macrophages, which produce substances that cause inflammation. Obesity can result in hypertension, hypercholesterolemia, diabetes, heart attacks, strokes, and even cancer. Chemical signals are Released by visceral fat. signals that interfere with metabolism and induce inflammation.

Obesity-related high blood pressure destroys stem cells and raises the risk of heart disease.

Excess body fat stresses cells and reduces insulin sensitivity, which is why type 2 diabetes and obesity are strongly related. Additionally, obesity has been linked to lower lung capacity, cognitive decline, and smaller brain size, all of which can result in breathing problems and organ damage. Obesity can lead to inflammation and blockage of the airways. Fat in the tongue and throat frequently causes sleep apnea, which causes headaches, fatigue, irritation, and problems learning. In addition, diabetes, heart attacks, heart failure, and strokes are all more likely to be caused by sleep apnea.

Additionally, obesity contributes significantly to the severity of COVID-19 since it increases Both inflammation and a weakened immune system.

The virus causes inflammation and damage to blood vessels throughout the body by specifically targeting fat cells. Additionally, obesity reduces lung function, which increases the body's susceptibility to respiratory infections like COVID-19. Individuals with obesity who recover from COVID-19 may have "long COVID," or persistent symptoms.

One of the several advantages of losing weight is a decrease in death rates.

Reducing weight, even by one to twenty pounds, can have a substantial positive impact on heart health by lowering blood pressure and heart failure risk. Significant weight loss can offer even greater advantages, such as lowering the chance of death from diabetes

Chapter 3

Maintaining a Sound Equilibrium

There are two forms of fat in the human body: visceral and subcutaneous. Visceral fat is found deep inside the body, whereas subcutaneous fat is the fat that may be pinched and emits hormones that have an impact on biological processes. Fat functions as an organ, releasing hormones, regulating metabolism, storing energy, and hunger, as well as reducing inflammation. Consequently, getting rid of the ultimate objective shouldn't be to rid oneself of all fat. Keeping a healthy weight and balancing a healthy weight are essential to general well-being. Underweight people must deal with comparable mortality risks to those who are overweight.

Additionally, fat is what triggers your body's adaptive thermogenesis mechanism. This implies that your body heats up as a result of fat. Brown fat generates heat and regulates body temperature. It is what provides warmth to animals who are hibernating in the cold.

3.1: Consume a diet high in fruits, veggies, and proteins that is well-balanced.

 A healthy diet may affect every aspect of your life, including how your body and brain work. At every meal, try to consume a balanced diet by avoiding processed sweets, consuming lots of lean protein, and covering half of your plate with fruits and vegetables.

• Aim for five servings or more of fruits and vegetables each day. This may contain everything from kale in a kale pesto sauce to smoothies and steaming vegetable sides.

Whenever feasible, choose whole grain and whole wheat items such as pasta, bread, and other starchy foods. These foods are higher in fiber and higher in vitamins and minerals.

• Eating a well-balanced diet does not always imply trying to reduce weight. You may still gain by making little dietary adjustments regularly, even if you are at a healthy weight. To begin, increase your daily intake of fresh vegetables to only one serving. You won't believe the impact that little adjustments may have on your diet. Before making significant dietary changes, always consult your physician. They can assist you in determining the healthiest diet for your requirements.

3.2 Engage in 150 minutes or more of exercise each week.

Try some other forms of exercise, such as swimming, dancing, running, walking, or playing sports, then choose a sport you like.

Recall that to maximize, you should work out at a fairly intense speed for cardio. This indicates that you can hardly carry on a conversation at the rate you're going.

• Hard work isn't necessary for successful exercise. Begin by going for a vigorous walk, dancing about your home, or engaging in any other enjoyable activity that causes your heart rate to rise. Even applications designed for total beginners are available.

• Strive to strength train each of the major muscle groups at least twice a week to maximize the benefits of your workout regimen. Lifting weights or performing bodyweight workouts like pushups and squats might help you manage this.

Exercise is an essential component of a healthy lifestyle since it makes your body robust and capable. Your body should be capable of handling the tasks you wish to do.

3.3 Sleep for seven to nine hours every night.

Create a nightly sleep schedule that you follow before going to bed. Establish a regular bedtime first. Disconnect from all devices around one hour before that time. Spend some time unwinding both physically and mentally, then change into cozy jammies and sleep. Your mind will be calmed and informed that you're getting better with this sort of regimen.

• Depending on your age, different sleep recommendations may apply. Be prepared to relax during the night.

It is advised that school-age youngsters sleep for nine to eleven hours per night. Teens require 8 to 10 hours per night, and seniors 65 and older require at least 7-8 hours. regular sleep schedule.

• Stay clear of bright displays an hour before bed. This covers televisions, computers, tablets, and phones. You could find it difficult to fall asleep because of the blue light from the screen.

Chapter 4

Mental well-being

4.1 Practice yoga, meditation, or self-massage to unwind your body.

It's critical to set aside some time each day for relaxation since mental stress can have a negative physical impact on your health. Indulging in yoga, meditation, a warm bath, or self-massage might aid in decompressing your body after a demanding day.

• Even though you have a lot of free time, consider setting aside just five minutes every day to help your body relax.

Try progressive muscle relaxation for a basic kind of relaxation. Shut your eyes, take a deep breath, and gradually tension your foot muscles for three counts. After that, let the muscles fully relax. Follow this sequence

Throughout your body, paying particular attention to your arms, shoulders, face, chest, legs, glutes, and core.

• Use applications to help you with meditation, such as Insight Timer or Headspace. These are excellent starting materials.

• Gaining more muscle via meditation enables you to respond and react more effectively to life's challenges.

4.2 Make attainable objectives that you may strive for each day.

Establishing short- and long-term objectives might assist you in organizing your actions and plans. Try putting one or two major life objectives on paper. Subdivide the objective into many more manageable objectives. Next, deconstruct those objectives into manageable actions.

• If being healthy is one of your objectives, for instance, you may have two smaller objectives: finishing a 5K and obtaining a 6-pack. To reach those objectives, you may then deconstruct each of them into a unique exercise regimen.

• Aim to maintain realistic goals. Dream big, but don't go out of your way to become the richest person on the planet. This is an ambitious objective that is unattainable for the great majority of individuals. Alternatively, consider establishing a goal, such as accumulating enough money for a house or a comfortable retirement.

• Keep a journal to help you stay focused on your objectives. You may write things down, consider them, and make changes to them from time to time when you use a diary.

4.3: Engage in a joyful activity each day.

Achieving and maintaining objectives can boost your self-esteem. Setting goals might potentially improve your emotional well-being. Every day, engage in an activity that makes you happy.

Every day, set aside some time to accomplish at least one activity that brings you joy. This can include engaging in a pastime, going out on the town with friends, spending time with your loved ones, or doing anything else that relieves you from the pressures of the day. If you don't already have a pastime that you love, consider taking up something new, such as dancing, creating, playing sports, or collecting items. Try to switch up a few enjoyable things that you enjoy doing. In this manner, you may continue to engage in your Pastime or watch your favorite show even if you are unable to go out with friends.

- It's okay to laugh at yourself while you're picking up new activities or simply making errors in life. whole person and you ought to have confidence in your innate value as a lovely, imperfect human being.

4.4: Acquire new knowledge.

Developing and stimulating your intellect is essential to maintaining mental wellness. Learn something new or gain more information on a subject you are interested in to keep your mind active. It doesn't take a lot of time to challenge your mind; some examples are learning a new language, reading for a certain amount of time each day, picking up a new instrument, or learning how to program. You can stay sharp by devoting even five minutes a day to learning something new.

4.5: Take care of your spiritual health.

If you consider yourself to be religious, set aside time in your calendar to practice your faith. This may be going to church once a week or praying every day.

offerings. Even if you don't practice religion, you could think about things like

Meditation or a stroll in the outdoors might help you stay centered and

centered on enjoying the now rather than stressing about what could come.

• Living a balanced existence does not require religious beliefs. Nonetheless, scheduling time for your faith should be a component of your balance if it is significant to you.

Chapter 5

Balancing work and life:

5.1: Create a budget for yourself.

A balanced existence requires sound financial management in addition to physical and mental health.

wellness. Begin simply by allocating funds for a budget that allows you to meet your present expenses.

of existence. After creating your budget, consider pursuing other financial objectives such as debt repayment, house purchases, or retirement savings.

• All of your cost-of-living expenses, such as rent or mortgage, utilities, groceries, automobile or transit pass payments, credit card and student loan payments, and any Other regular costs, should be included in your budget.

• Little adjustments to your finances might add up. By the end of the year, you may lower your obligations by an additional $260 by investing just $5 every week. If you are having trouble organizing your money, you might want to try tracking your expenditures and creating a budget with a free tool like Mint. You may also check into taking a financial planning or budgeting course at your neighborhood community center.

5.2: Try to minimize the amount of work you accomplish at home.

Maintaining a physical separation between your home and professional lives can

support the maintenance of a good work-life balance. Aim to retain your employment, including

Anything from your workplace, including your business computer and papers, away from your private residence.

• Establish separate areas for work and home if you work from home or telecommute. For example, you may set aside a bedroom as your workplace. If so, don't keep your business computer open on the dining room table; instead, leave it in your office.

• When you get home from work, try to disconnect your electronics. Refrain from answering business calls. Take time to engage in non-computer hobbies such as cooking, reading, or creating.

5.3 Establish limits with your social groups, both at work and at home.

It is crucial to express when you are and aren't accessible to tackle work-related matters, even if your schedule is flexible. If you cannot or will not reply by 3 a.m., let your supervisor and coworkers know. SMS requesting a report by six in the morning.

• During the working day, your social groups ought to have a comparable boundary. Let them know that your job is your primary responsibility from 8 a.m. to 5 p.m., or whenever you work. If you want to talk during the workday, catch up with them at lunch or during a break. By the same token, you can reserve specified periods for activities unrelated to work. For example, if you run every day, you may set aside 7 to 8 a.m. as your running window. Don't read business emails at that time; instead, focus on enjoying your exercise.

5.4 If you need to renegotiate your job responsibilities, speak with your office.

If you're finding it challenging to maintain the work-life balance you want because of your employment,

wish, discuss new terms with your HR representative or supervisor. Things you might bring up options like modifying your hours to better meet your schedule or working one or two days a week from home.

• You don't have to give too much information but be ready to explain why your request is necessary. Most employers won't arbitrarily change your timetable. When you have to pick up your child from daycare, they could be more accommodating to your working a different schedule.

• It could be time to look for new work if you realize that your current one is too demanding or rigid to allow you to take care of your family or yourself. Seek accommodations that Provide the level of flexibility necessary to enable you to effectively manage your everyday schedule.

• If you don't feel the best about your job, consider the reasons behind it, as they may point to areas where you may feel better about it. For example, going out for coffee with your coworkers can help you feel more connected to them, and asking for greater autonomy when working on a project might help you feel more creative.

• Assign work to others when you can. Have faith in coworkers and associates to assist with significant initiatives. To lessen the load at home, divide up the responsibilities among family members.

Chapter 6

Feeling fabulous

You are amazing! You truly are; that much is true. I do not mean the concept of the ego or the delusion of being amazing. I refer to your entire being, including your body, essence, heart, and soul. You are a spiritual entity going through a human transformation. This indicates that pure, loving, good energy is your source. This indicates that you are a pure, positive source of energy in physical form.

What is being fabulous?

Your intrinsic value, beauty, goodness, sensuality, passion, kindness, compassion, love, and joy are all part of who you are. It is believing in the Source and oneself. It's giving up. It's a way to recognize all the virtues and ideals you brought into this life.

Every day, love and joy flood your life when you live fully in your fabulousness.

You become a powerful magnet once you accept how amazing you are. A lady or guy who genuinely lives up to her fabulousness is loved by both sexes.

Men and women want to spend a lot of time with you when you know and radiate it. They don't give a damn about your age, size, or attire.

6.1: What Obstructs the Feeling of Fabulousness?

The voice of the ego or self-criticism gets in the way.

Silencing the ego that berates you is the first step toward comprehending how amazing you are. It is impossible to feel wonderful when you give in to ANY self-criticism. Therefore, whether you make fun of your legs, your Education, or your background, you are denying yourself of your amazing potential because of your lack of attendance at that institution, your level of enthusiasm, etc.

Why would you act in such a way? Is it customary? Because it seems familiar, because so many women, do it? since you believe the criticisms to be accurate?

They are all falsehoods, after all. Any self-criticism is self-deception.

You might wish to make some changes to some aspects of yourself. Great if you can accomplish it right now. Modify them. Go ahead and do whatever it is you want to do—lose weight, get it back, learn to sing or dance, tone your muscles, etc.

6.2: Quit whining and start doing something.

It costs a fortune to complain. Hatred is the price. I did that for years, so I know. I also had to learn to quit berating myself once I stopped

having previously condemned myself. Oh, how cunning and vicious the ego can be! Thankfully, my spirit and compassion prevailed over my ego.

Furthermore, never expect a guy to support you in moving past your critiques. It's not their job, they can't do it, and they don't know how. You own it.

6.3: Recall: quit being critical of yourself.

It is keeping love away from you.

All the love and happiness you had when you were a newborn is still there in your heart and spirit; you just lost touch with it at some point. Regaining contact with it doesn't require much labor, but you must be prepared to put in some effort.

It's necessary to focus on the physical, mental, and spiritual aspects of your existence. needs to be addressed to feel amazing.

Bonus

Ten Everyday Actions to Boost Your Self-Esteem and Life

You should follow these instructions to get long-lasting benefits. They're easy and basic. You will be pleased with the outcome.

1. Begin each day with five minutes of appreciation before you get out of bed.

Identify three things that make you smile. You may be thinking of anything—your new shoes, your pet, a close buddy, or even just your comfortable bed.

2. Go through three to five pages of a book that inspires you.

3. Exercise throughout the day. Every day. Even if it's simply stretching in front of the television, do something. Make a physical movement. Play some music, then spend ten minutes dancing. Move your body to Experience physical Play some music, then spend ten minutes dancing. Move with your body.

4. Consume wholesome meals and, most of all, consume modest quantities slowly. People frequently ask me why I'm so thin. I'll make you feel well physically. Increase to at least 30 minutes each day. Consume everything I want, even if it means having a cookie every

day, but I never overeat. Recall that food is fuel, and you require it for daily survival. Breakfast is important since it provides you with energy for the first portion of the day. You won't overeat at lunch or indulge in sugary snacks as a result.

5. Take some quiet time during the day. Meditation is the best option as it allows you to release the barriers that your mind constructs. Play a calming CD on your Headphones and allow yourself permission to unwind for ten to fifteen minutes.

6. Put on attire that makes you feel amazing. Give away any clothing that doesn't make you feel amazing and don't wear it. Have you ever noticed that you almost always bring your favorite outfits on vacation and very never bring something you don't like? Thus, avoid wearing those outfits at home. 7. Use Abraham's concentration wheel technique, which you may learn from his books, once a

day to change your negative ideas. It's a really powerful method for assisting you in changing a negative mindset to a positive one. It's both clever and easy. I'll mention it in the section on resources.

8. After that, make sure you show love to someone every day—it might be your partner, lover, friend, neighbor, cat, or dog. You will Enter the loving awareness as a result. It's essential for your spirit and heart.

9. Moreover, love yourself every day. Just picture yourself surrounding yourself with love energy in every cell of your body and heart.

10. Conclude your day with gratitude, just as you began it, before turning in for the night. Before you go to sleep, take a few minutes to express your gratitude for the day.

I promise that if you follow through on all of these actions for a full 30-day period, your self-perception will drastically change. You're going to feel amazing soon.

After three months, you won't even be able to recognize yourself; you'll feel like a goddess or God. Just picture yourself feeling amazing as you begin 2024. When January 1, 2024, arrives, you will look back on tonight and feel wonderful about yourself because you started doing everything I suggested.

9 798887 407081